Getting Ready for™ My Endoscopy

An Endoscopy Book for Kids – Preparation and Recovery

This book belongs to:

Written by Dr. Fei Zheng-Ward   Illustrated by Moch. Fajar Shobaru

Copyright © 2026 Fei Zheng-Ward

All rights reserved. Published by Fei Zheng-Ward, an imprint of FZWbooks. No part of this book may be copied, reproduced, recorded, transmitted, or stored by any means or in any form, electronic or mechanical, without obtaining prior written permission from the copyright owner.

Identifiers: ISBN 979-8-89318-147-0 (eBook)
 ISBN 979-8-89318-148-7 (paperback)
 ISBN 979-8-89318-149-4 (hardcover)

An endoscopy is a special test that helps your doctor take a careful look inside your food pipe, stomach, and part of your small intestine. Your doctor uses an endoscope, a soft, bendy tube with a tiny camera and light inside, to help them see.

The tube moves gently, like a soft noodle or spaghetti.

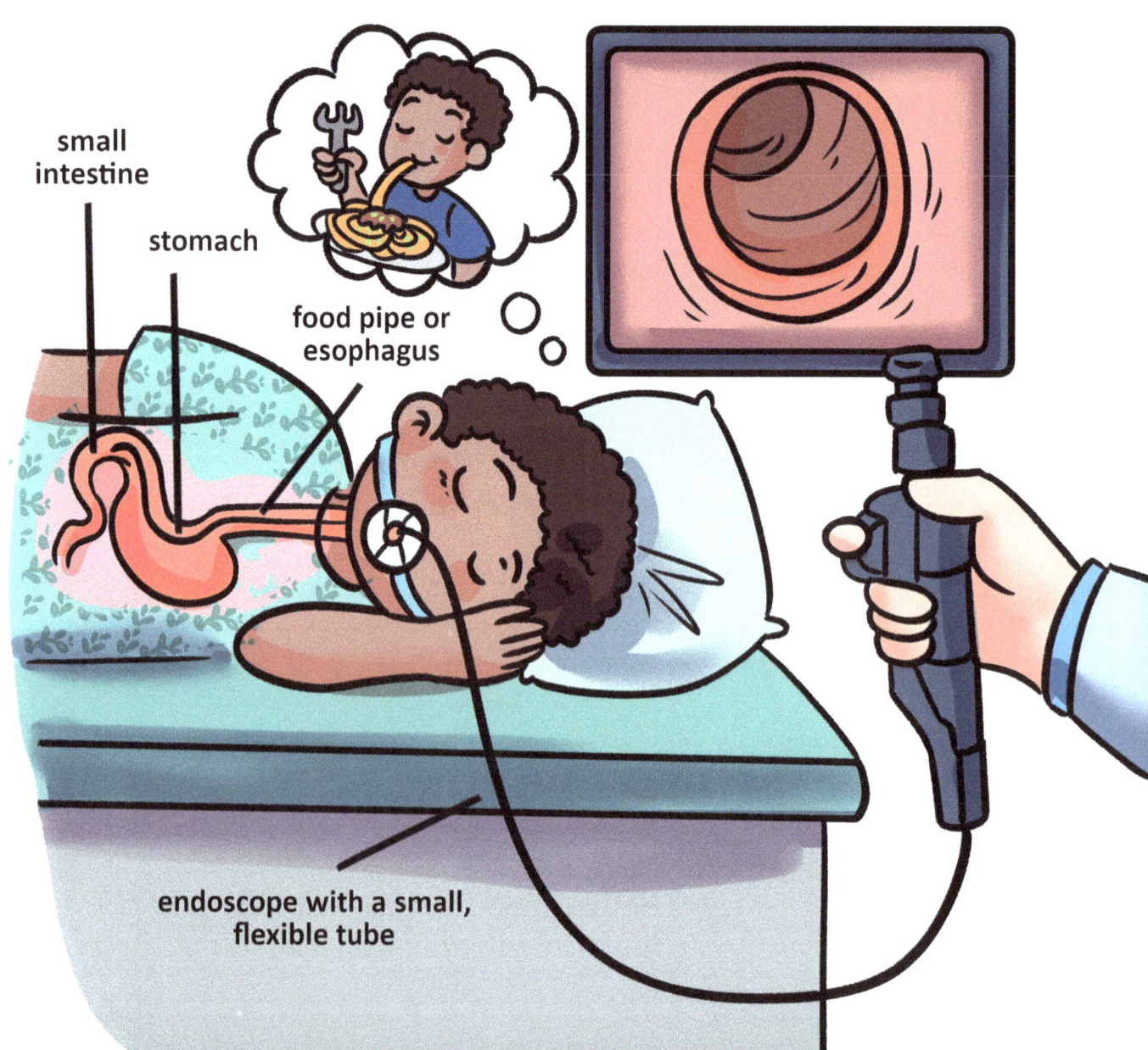

Check the box that shows why you need this test.

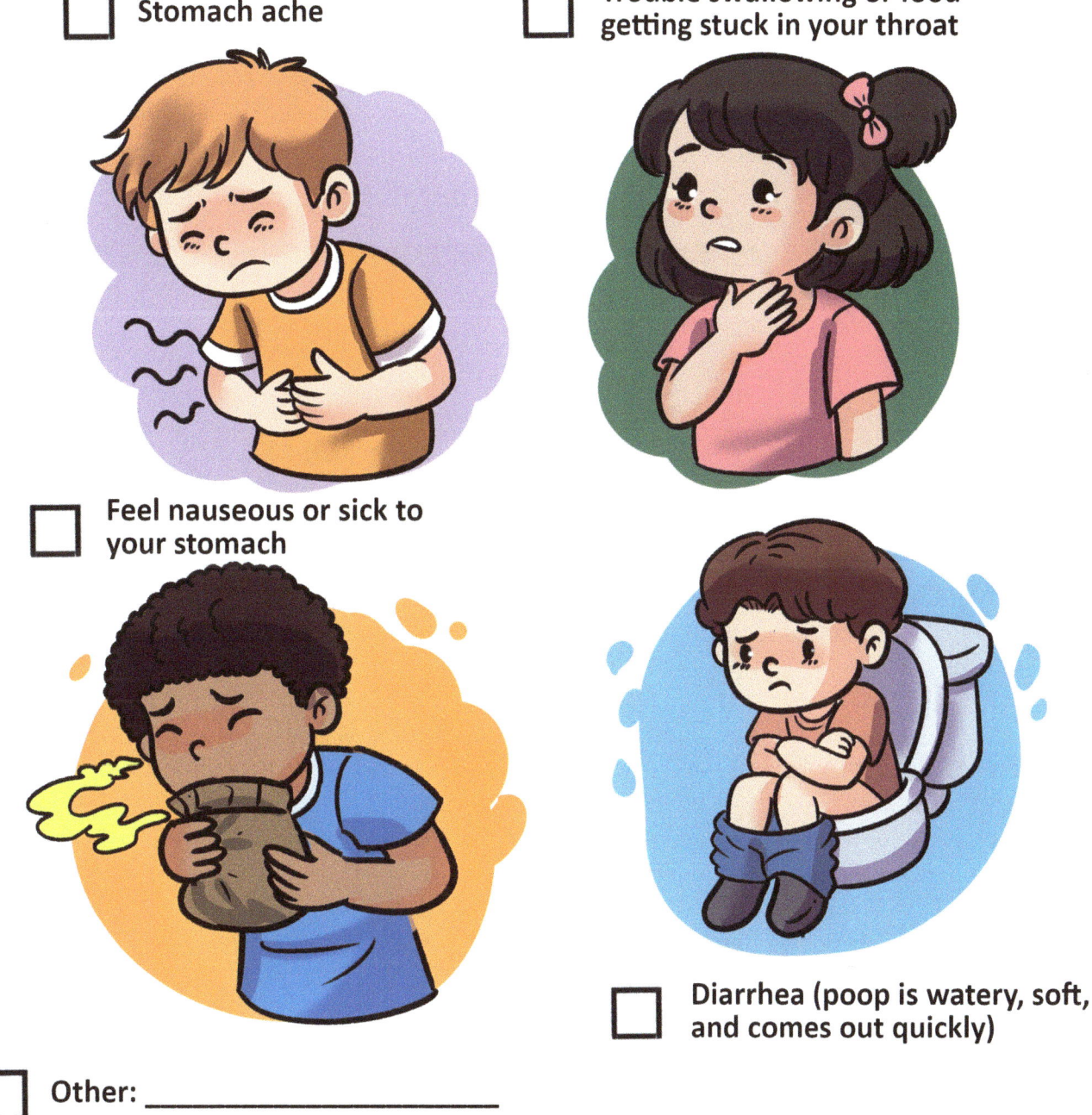

- ☐ Stomach ache
- ☐ Trouble swallowing or food getting stuck in your throat
- ☐ Feel nauseous or sick to your stomach
- ☐ Diarrhea (poop is watery, soft, and comes out quickly)
- ☐ Other: _____

On the day of your endoscopy,
you will skip breakfast and arrive at the hospital.

You might feel a little nervous—and that's okay.

You can bring your
favorite toy or blanket.

You can do this!

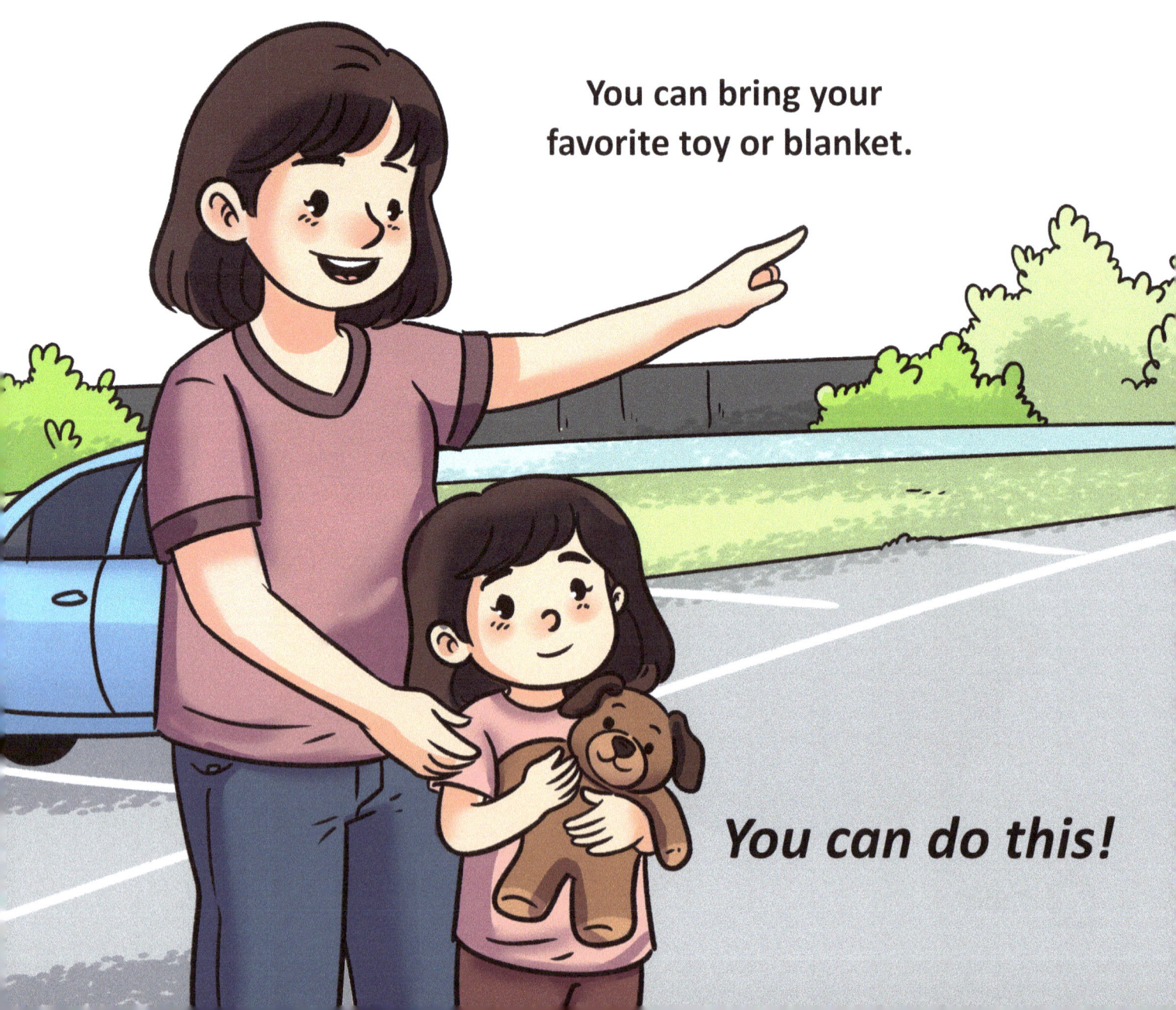

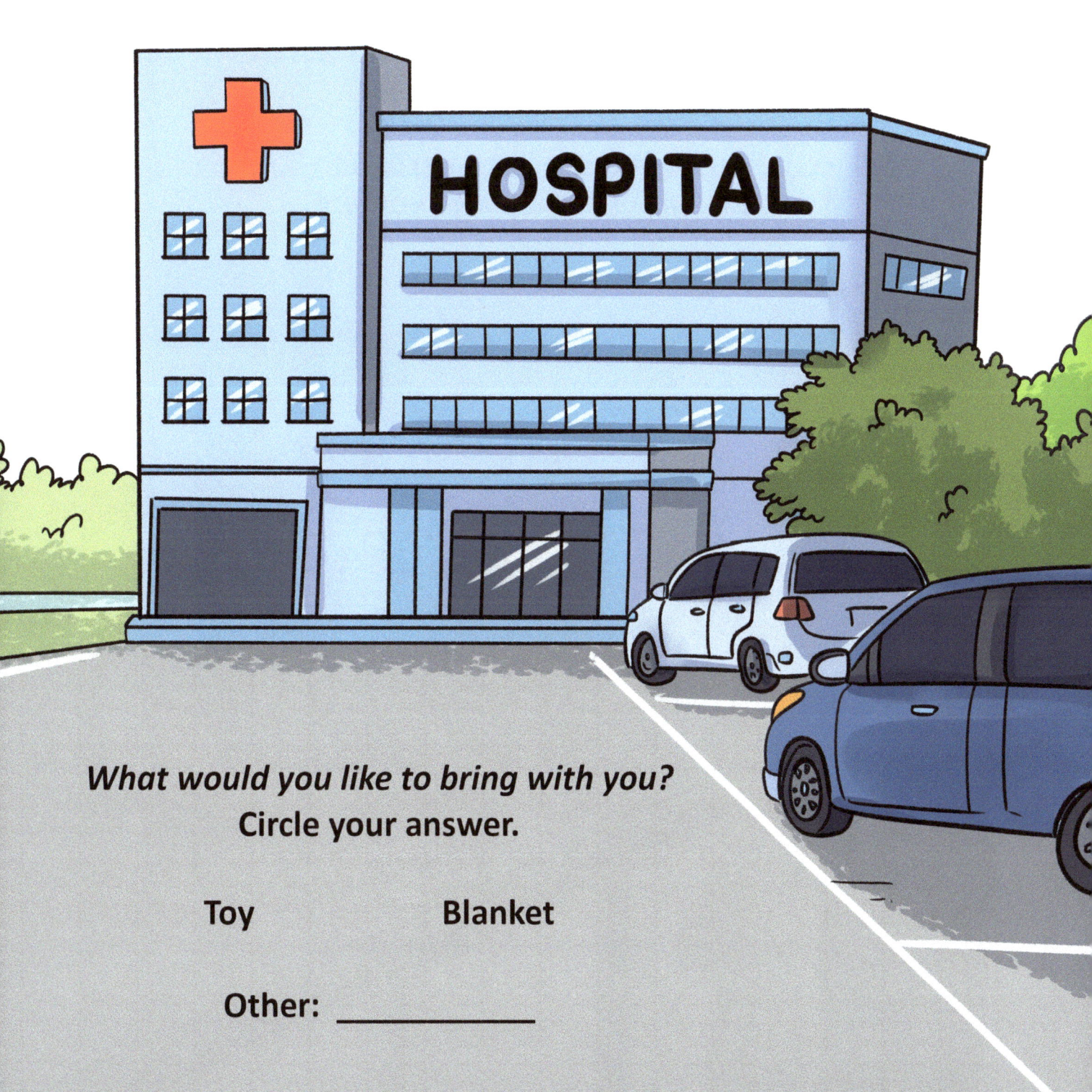

**What would you like to bring with you?
Circle your answer.**

Toy   Blanket

Other: _____

When you arrive, you'll check in and tell them your name and birthday.

You'll get a special wristband so everyone knows who you are.

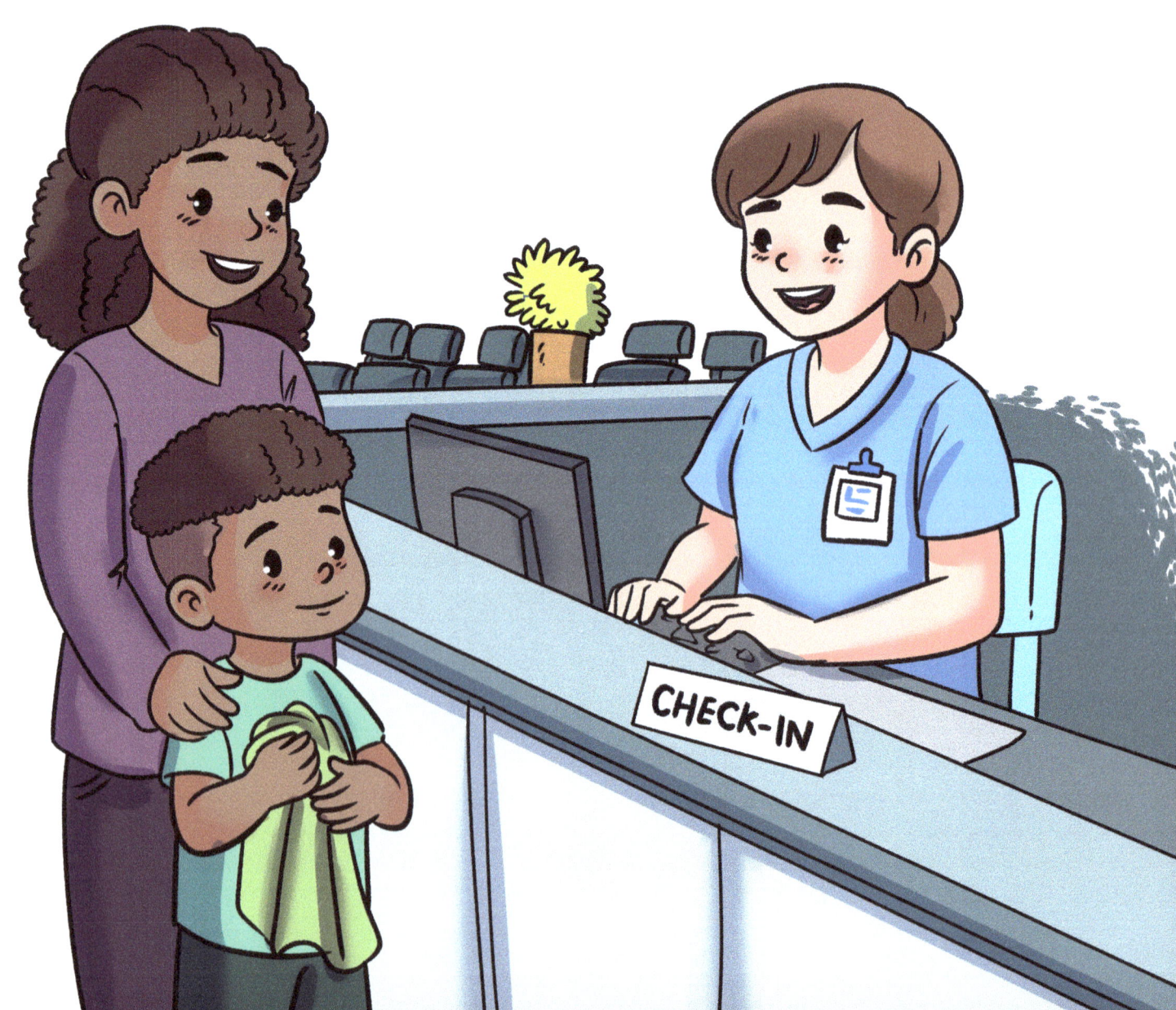

What color wristband will you get?
Circle the color of <u>your</u> wristband below.

Red   Green   Yellow

Blue   Pink   Orange

Purple   Black   White

Other: _____

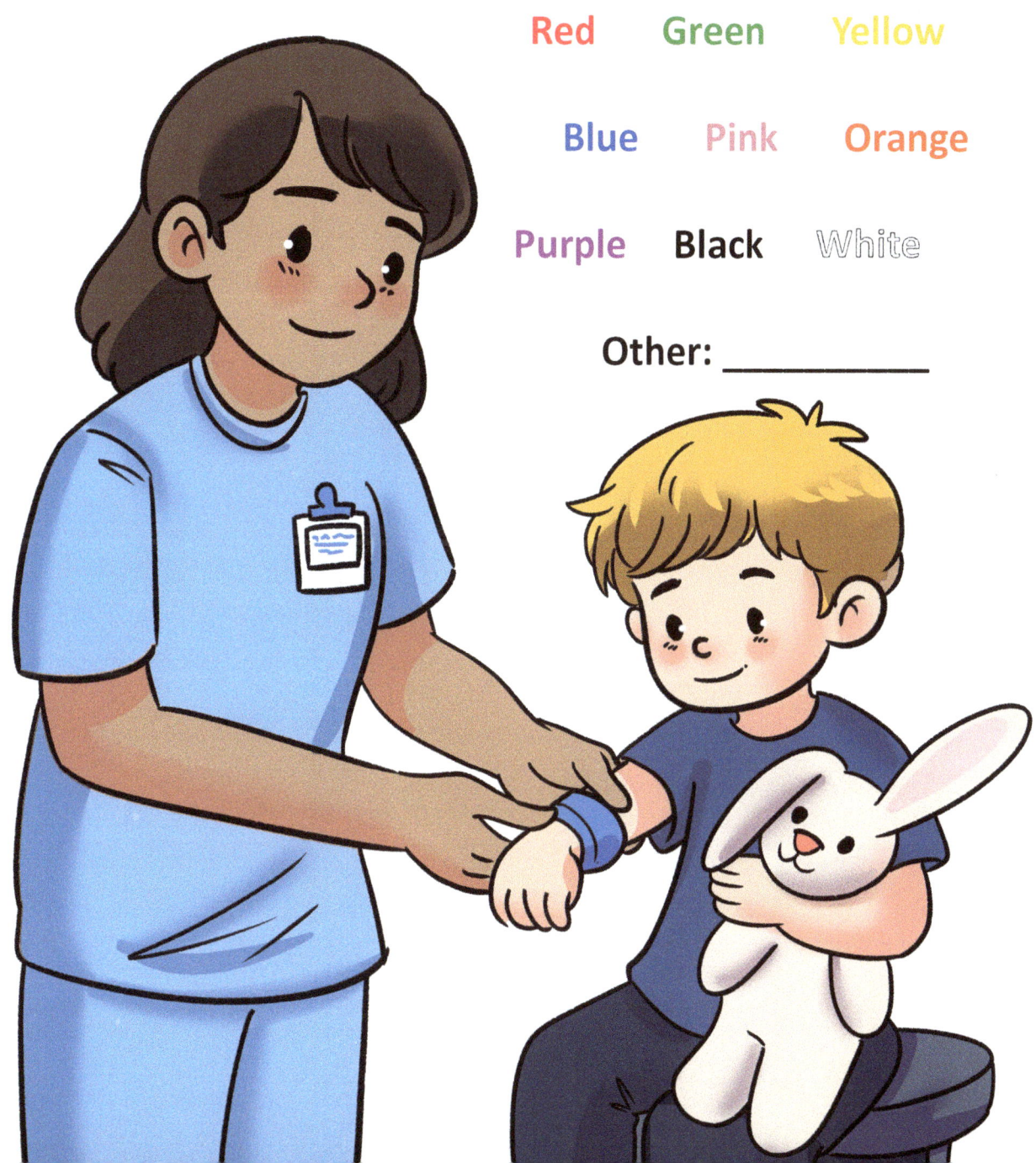

They will check your weight and height.

Do you know how much you weigh?

Do you know how tall you are?

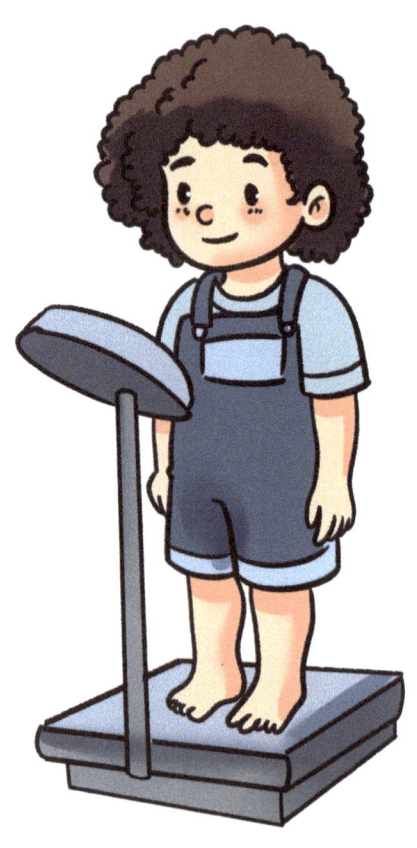 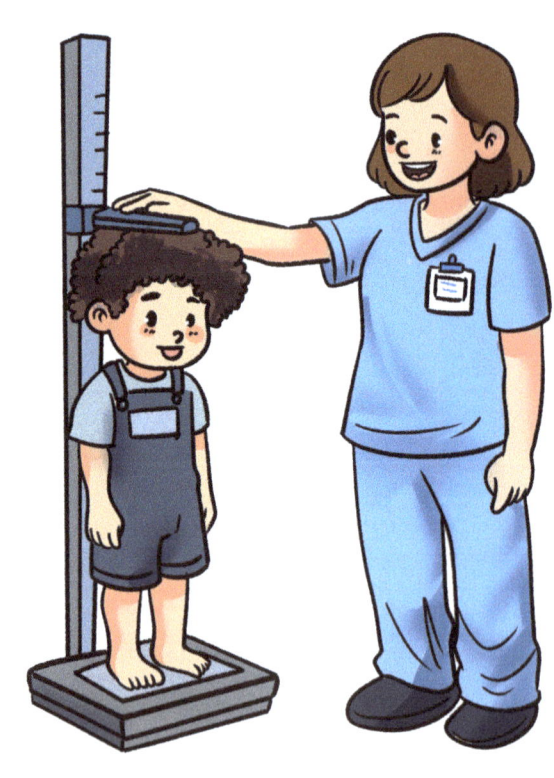

My weight is: _____   **My height is: _____**

You will change into a new outfit, put on a hat, a gown (it's like a backward superhero cape!), and some cozy socks.

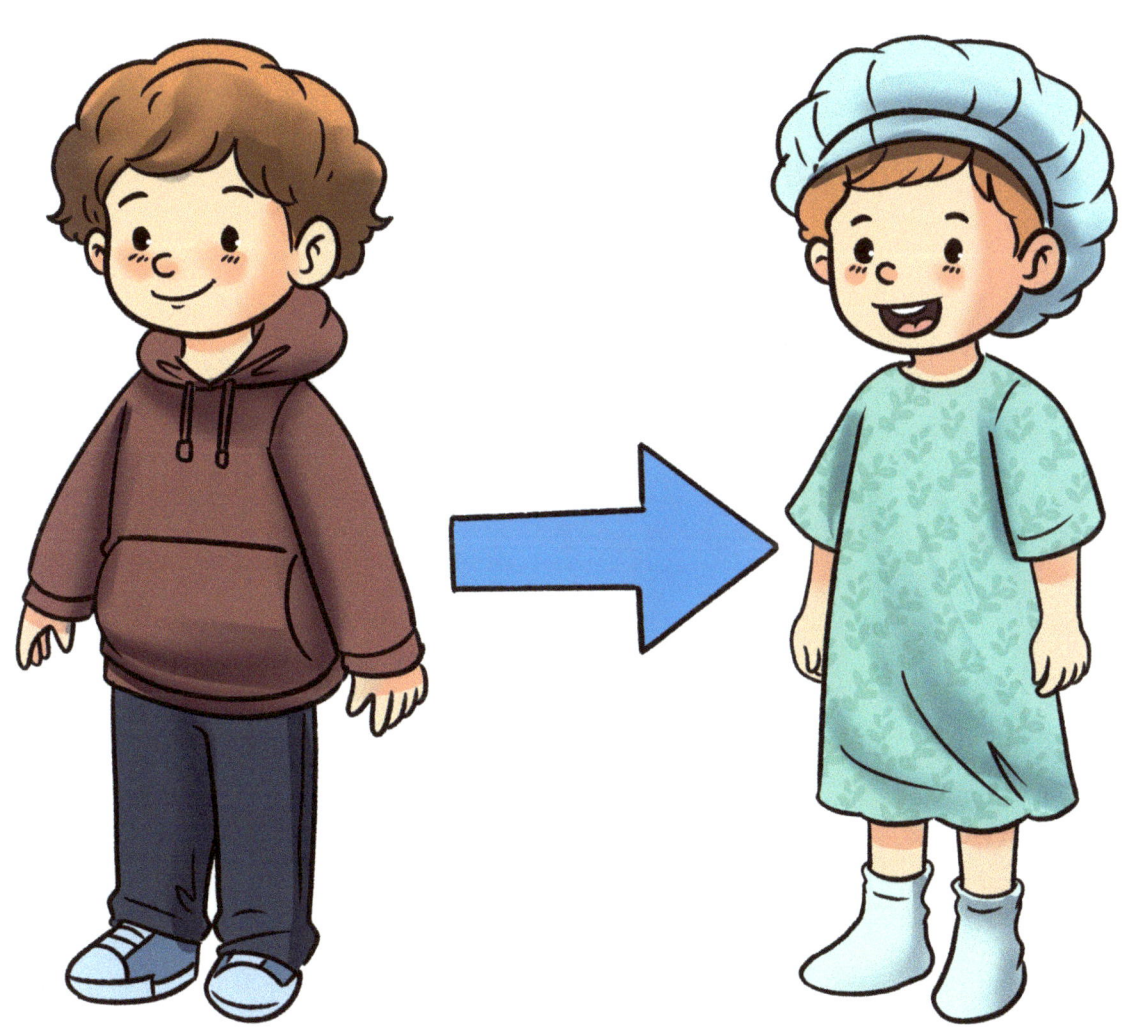

You've got this!

Your nurse will use a small tool called a pulse oximeter (or pulse ox) to see how much oxygen is in your body.

Oxygen comes from the air you breathe. It helps you move, play, and grow!

Which finger or toe do you want to use?

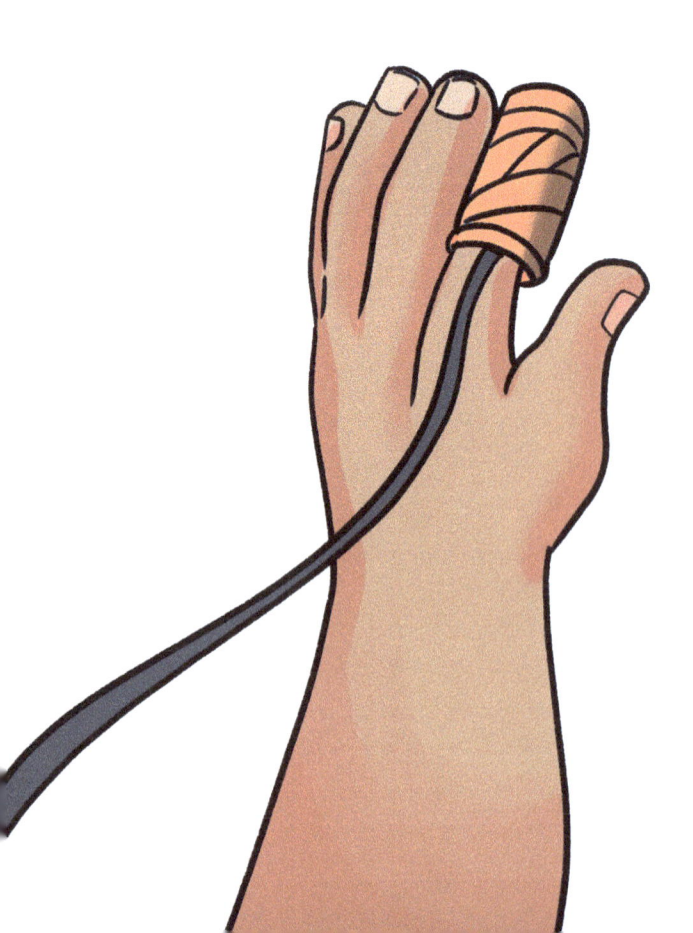
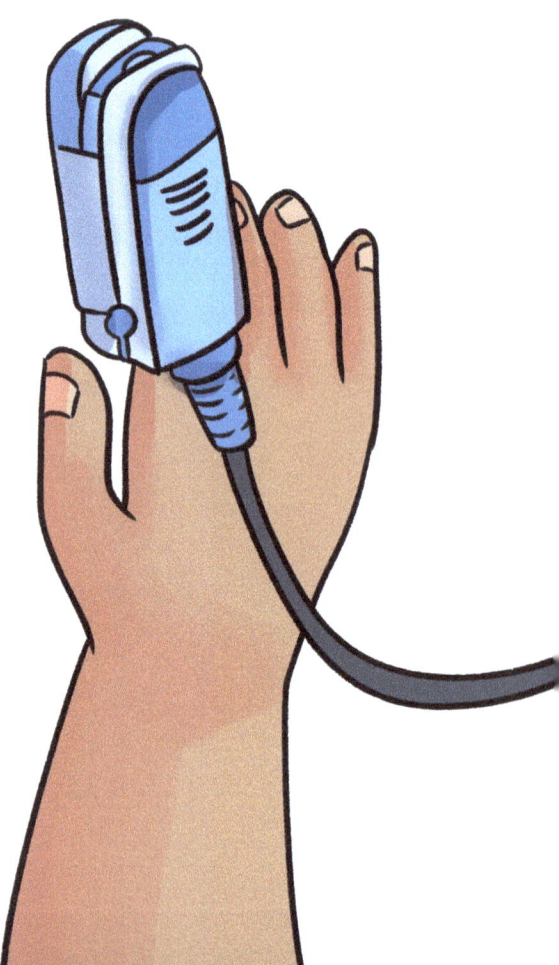

Your nurse or doctor may listen to your heart and lungs.

You'll get a blood pressure cuff around your arm or leg.
It will give you a BIG hug!
Try to stay still.

Are you ready?

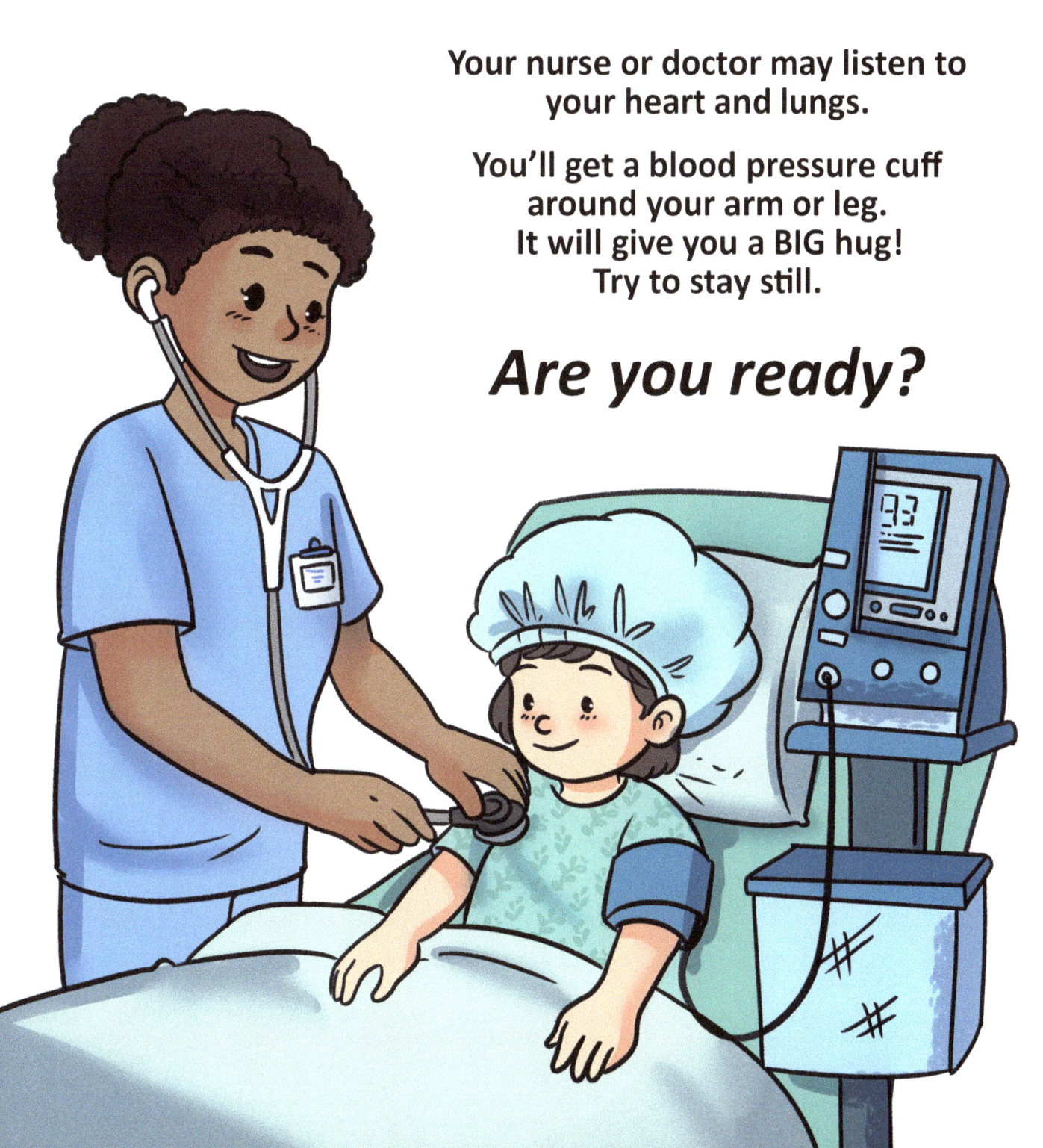

Are you feeling nervous or a little scared?
That's okay.

You may get a special medicine that helps your body feel calm and relaxed.

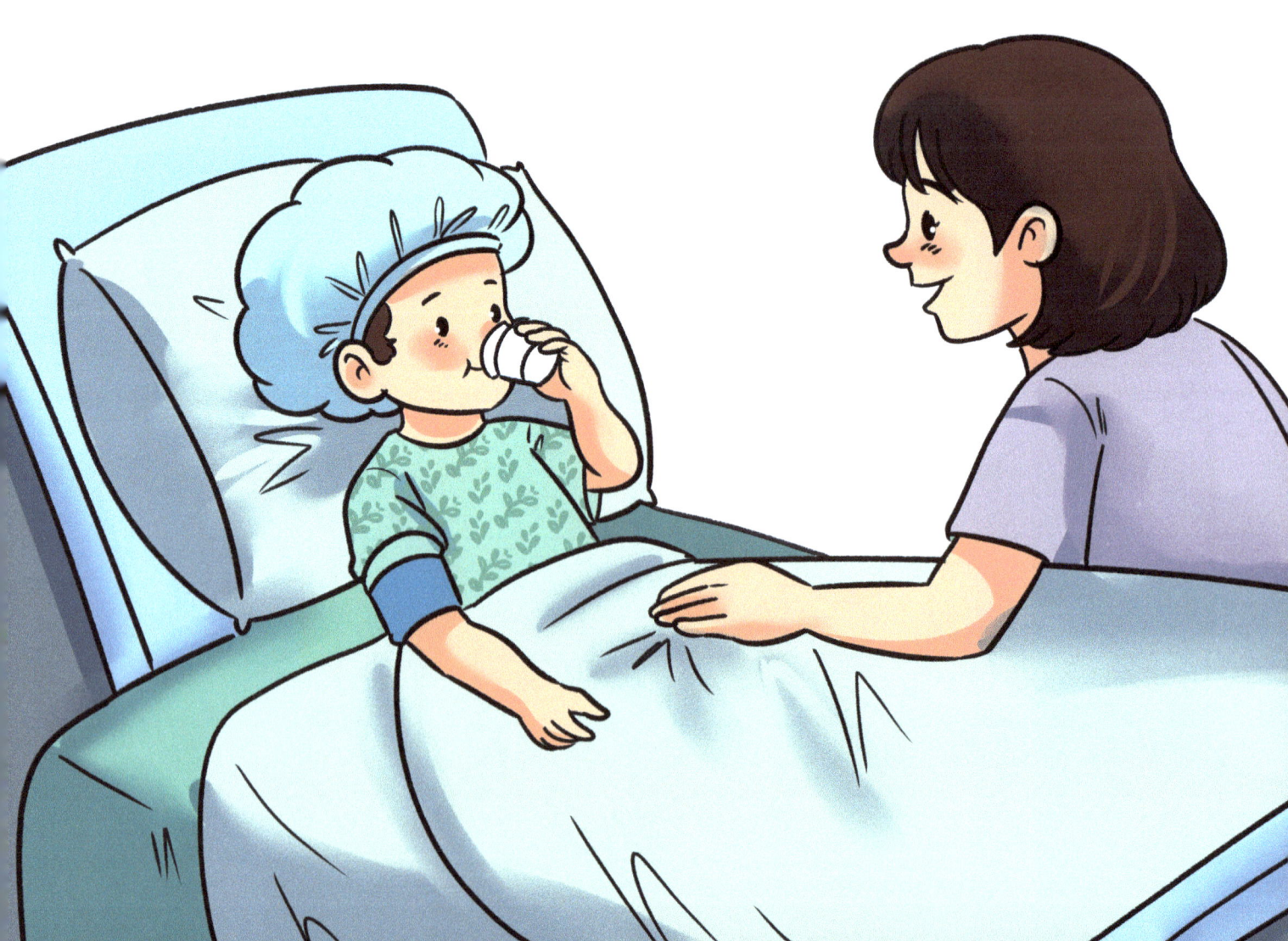

Your friendly nurses and doctors will come say hello and take good care of you.

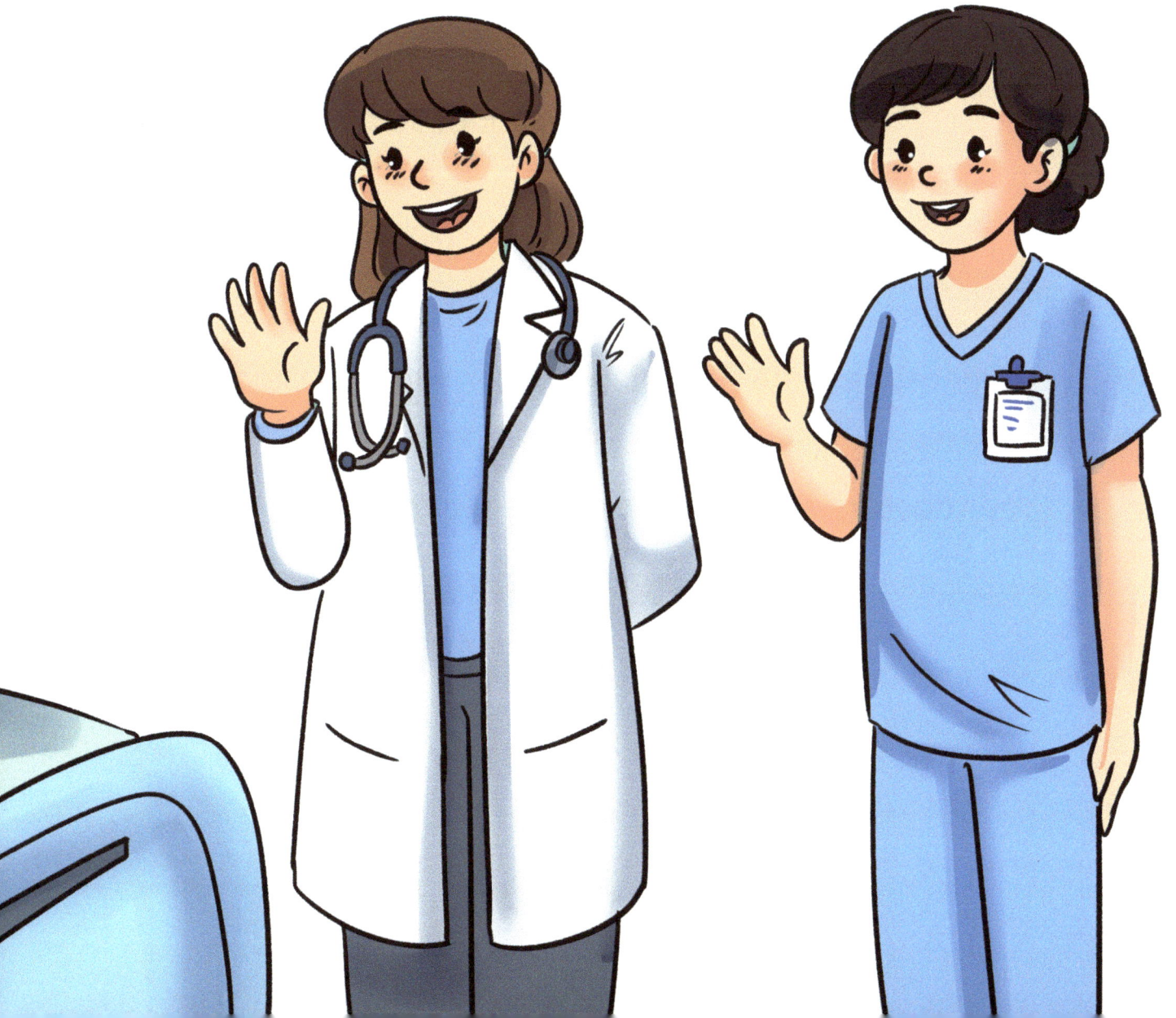

You will need an IV for your endoscopy.
It's a tiny straw that gives your body medicine.

Sometimes it is placed before you fall asleep.
It may feel like a quick poke.
Before it is placed, numbing cream can be used to help your skin feel more comfortable.

Other times, the IV is placed after you are asleep.

Your doctors and nurses will choose the safest way.

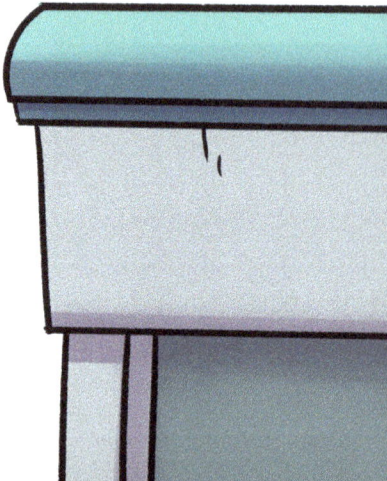

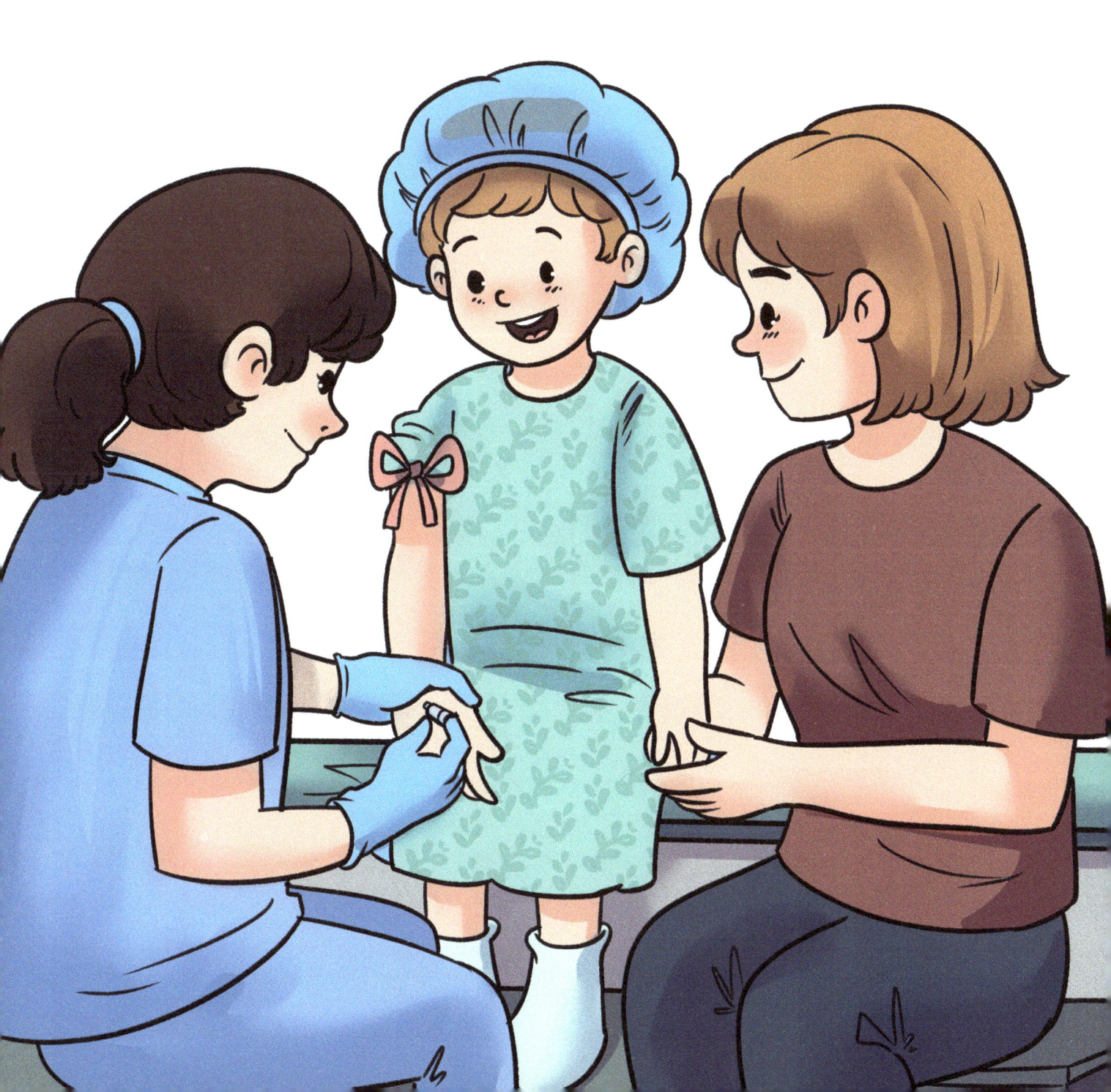

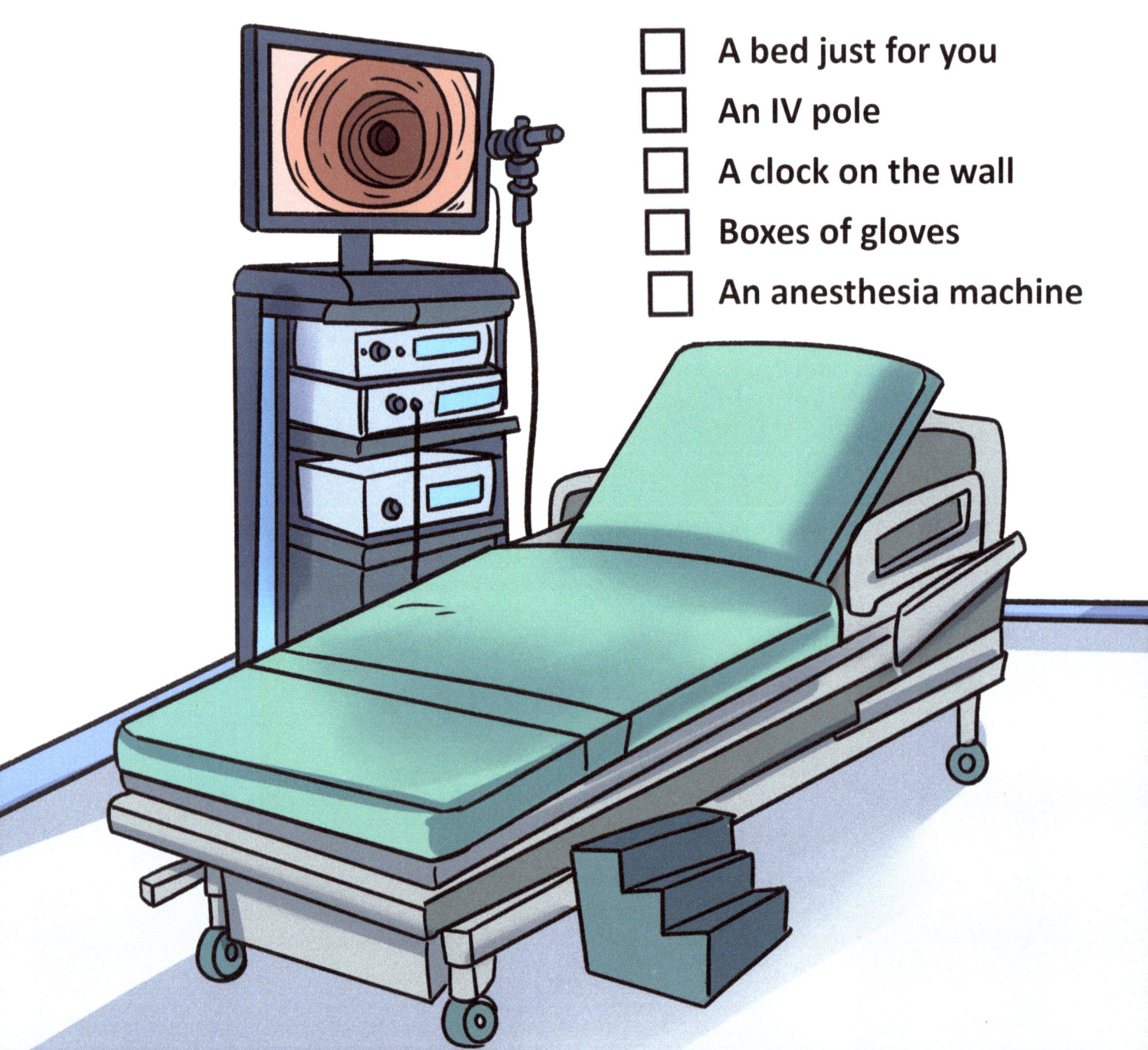

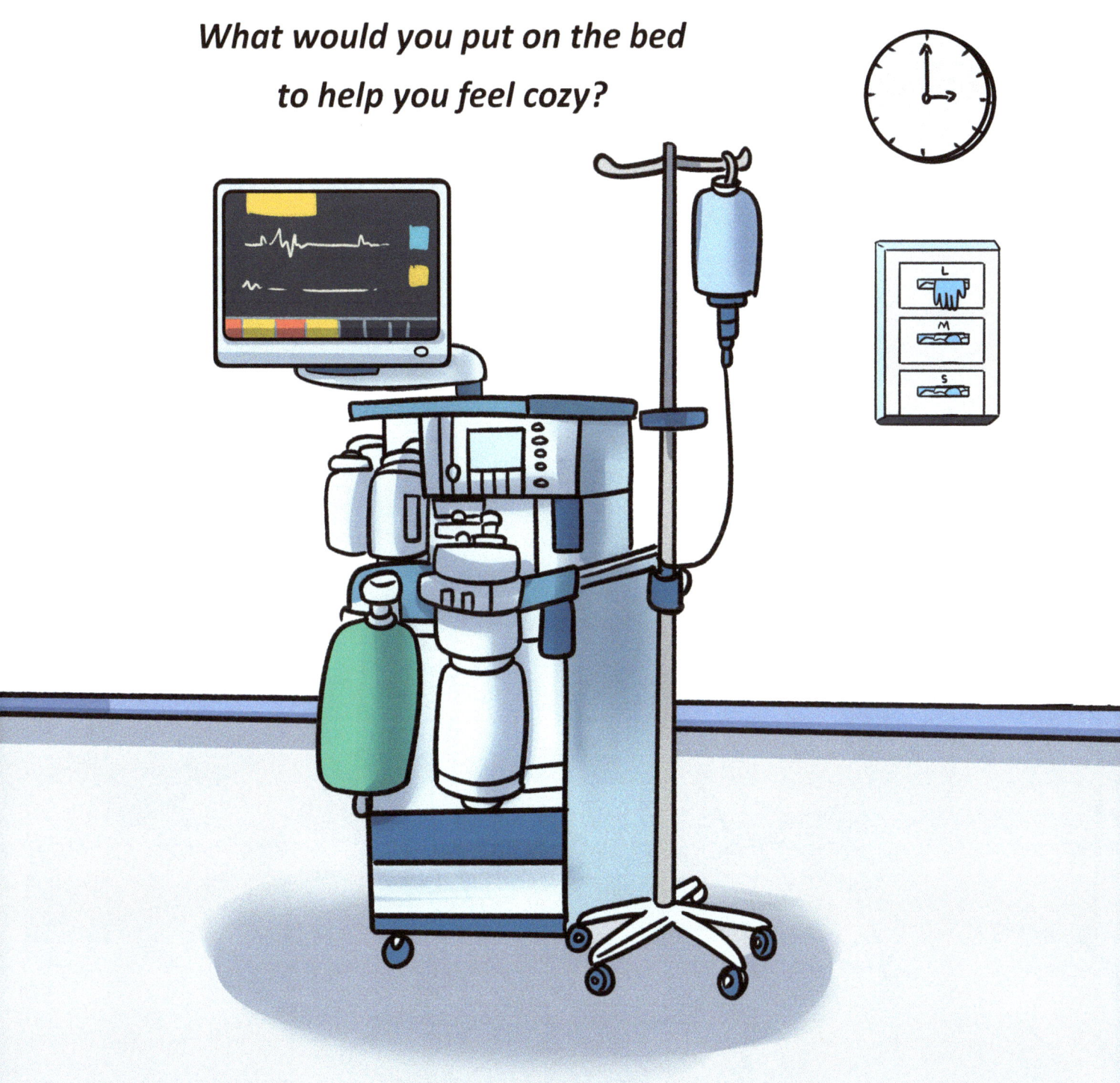

To help you fall asleep, you may get medicine through your IV...

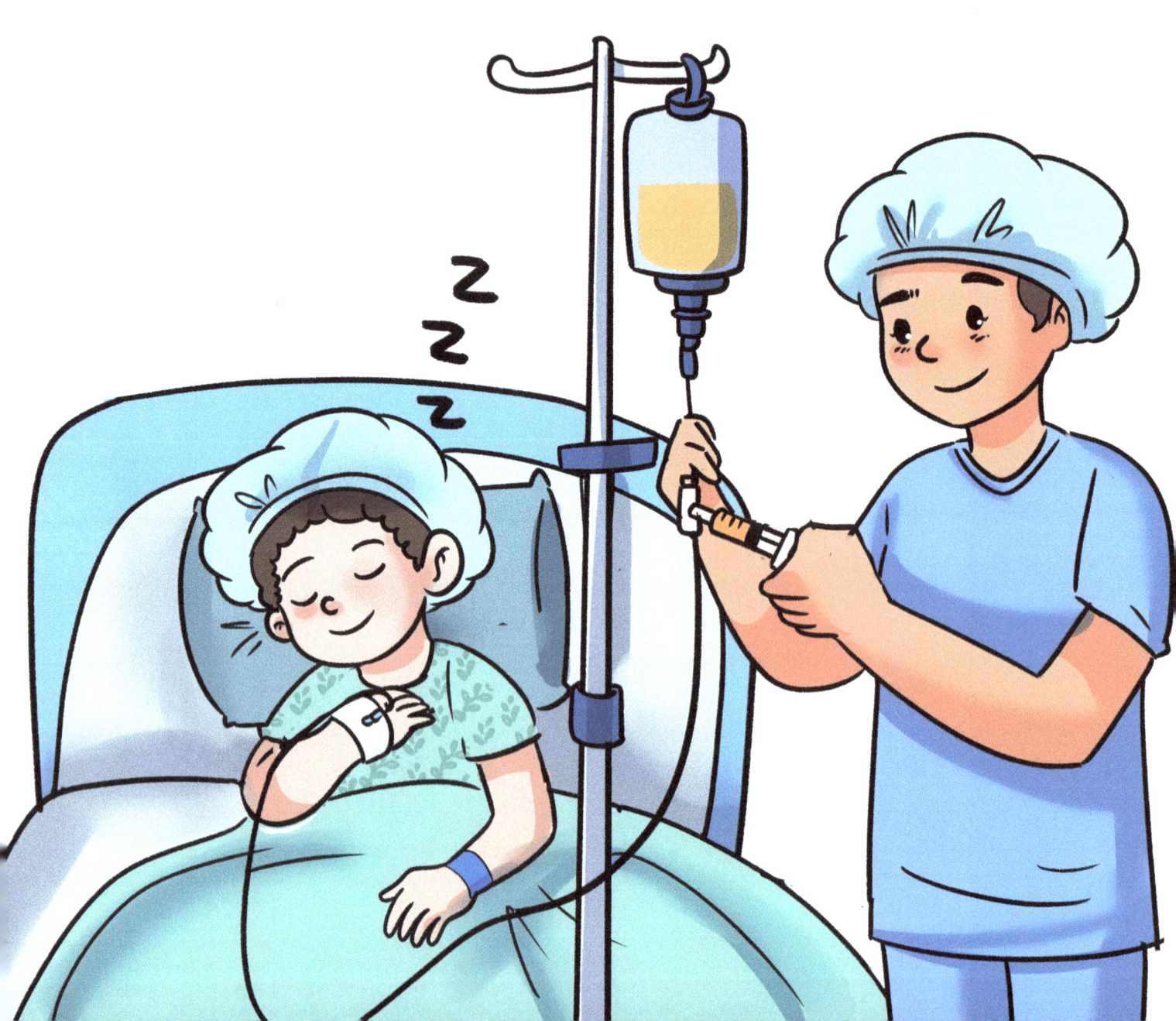

Or you may breathe sleepy air through a soft mask.

Your care team will decide which way is best and safest for you.

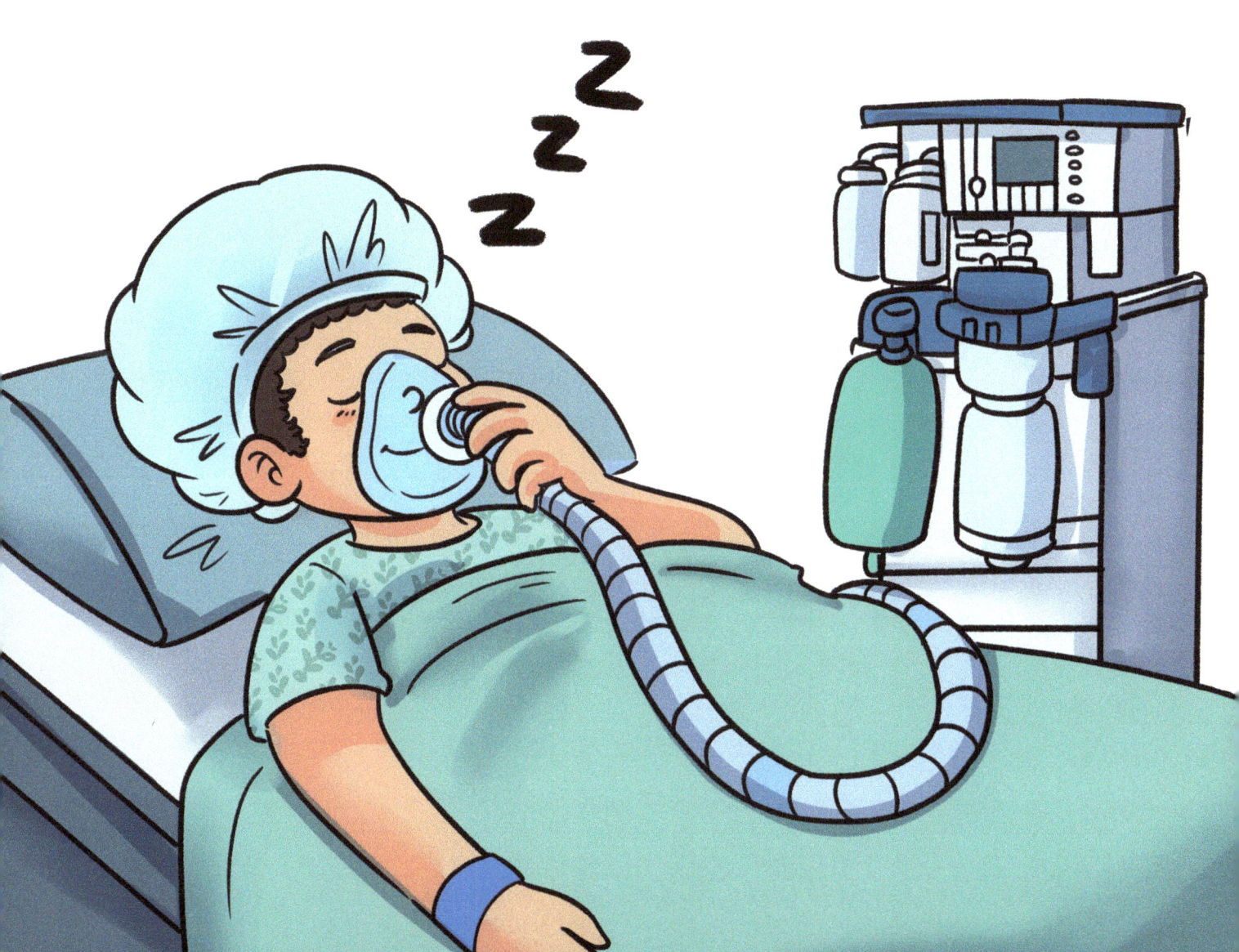

While you sleep and dream, your doctor gently uses the endoscopy camera to take a look inside.

The test is quick, and you won't feel a thing!

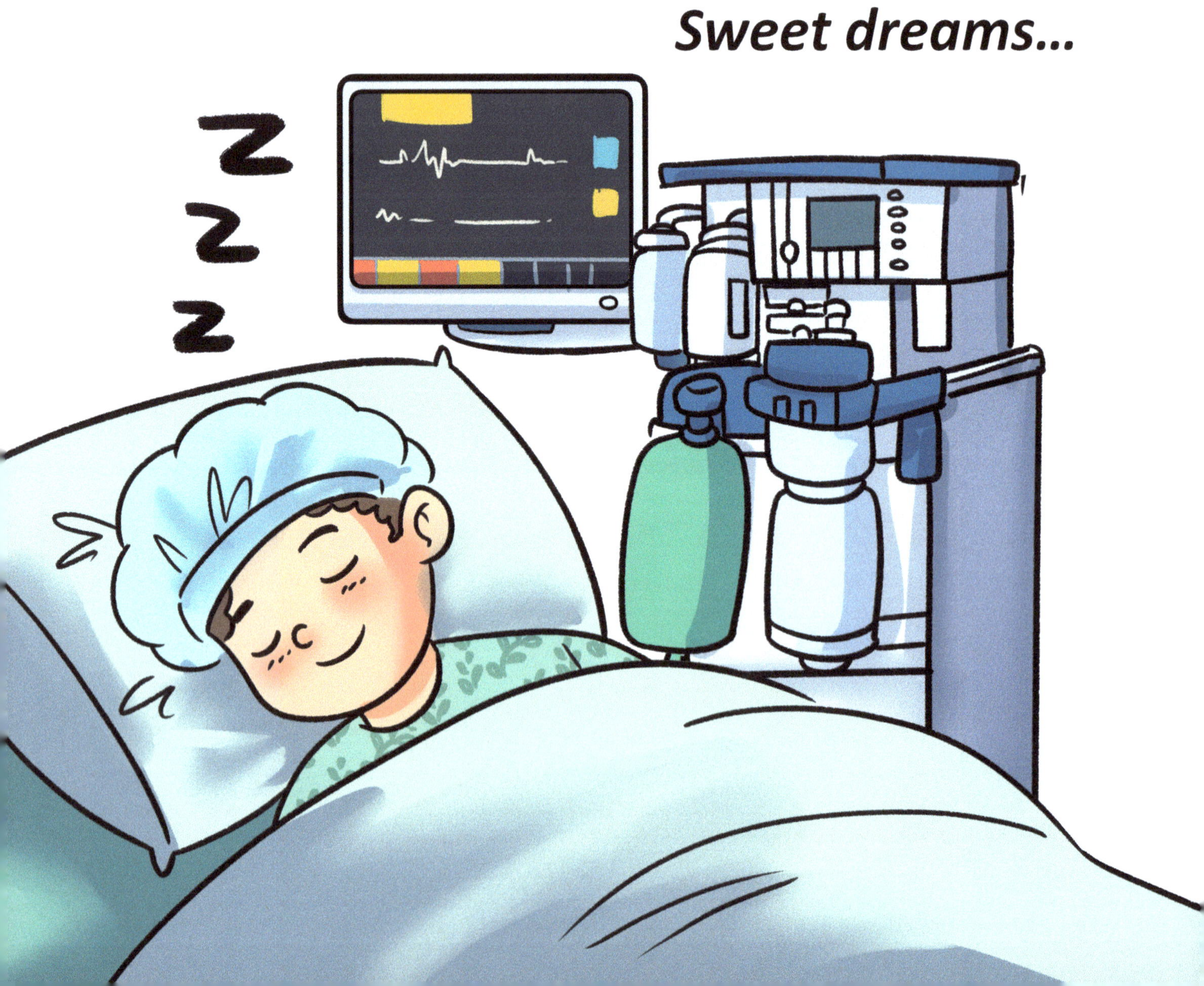

Sweet dreams...

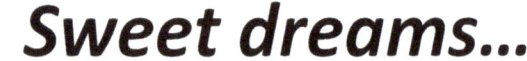

Your nurses and doctors will keep you safe and comfortable the whole time.

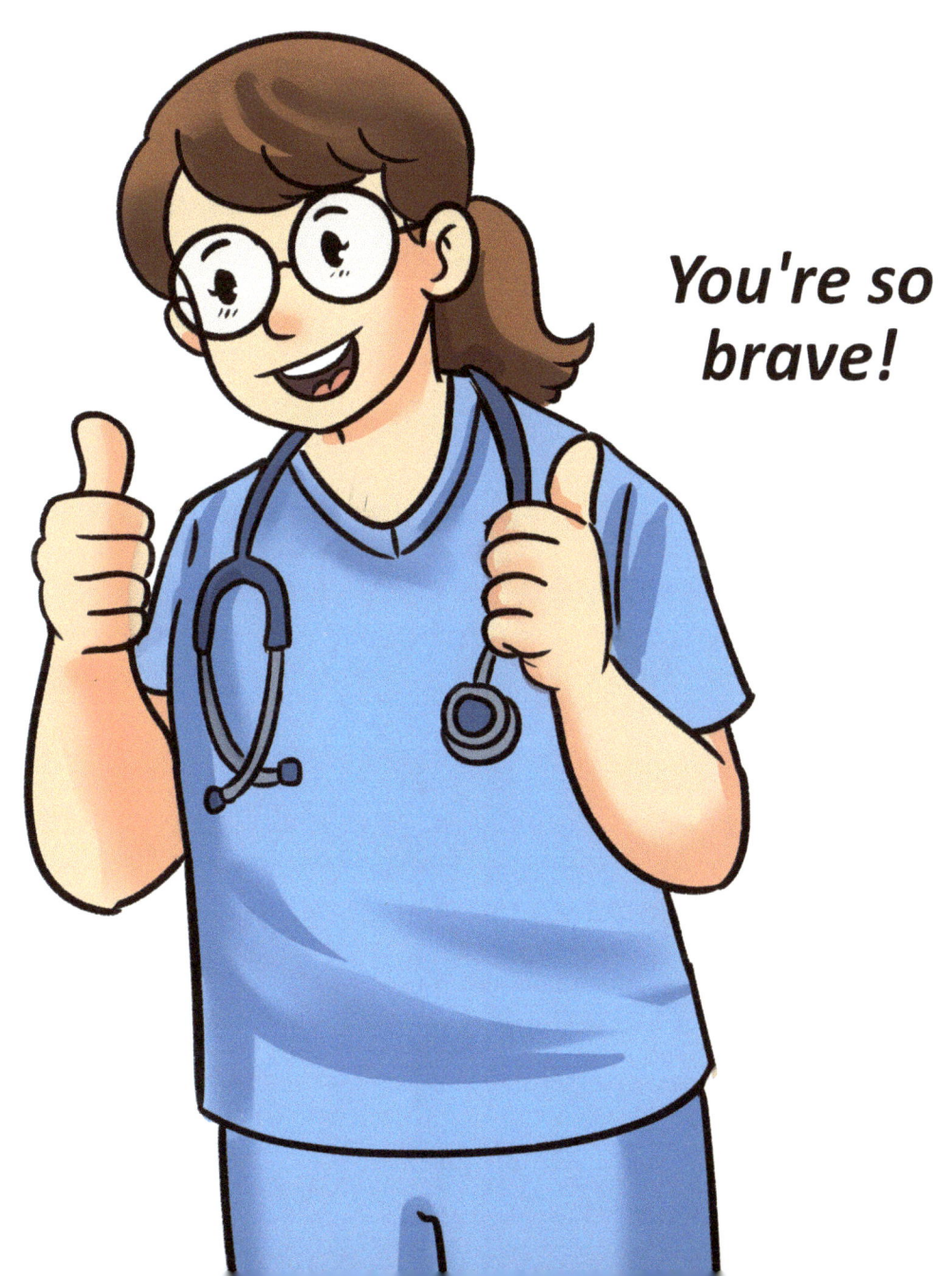

You're so brave!

When you wake up, you may have a sore throat, a belly ache, or feel sleepy or tired.

You may also feel like burping or passing gas (farting) from below.

That's normal!

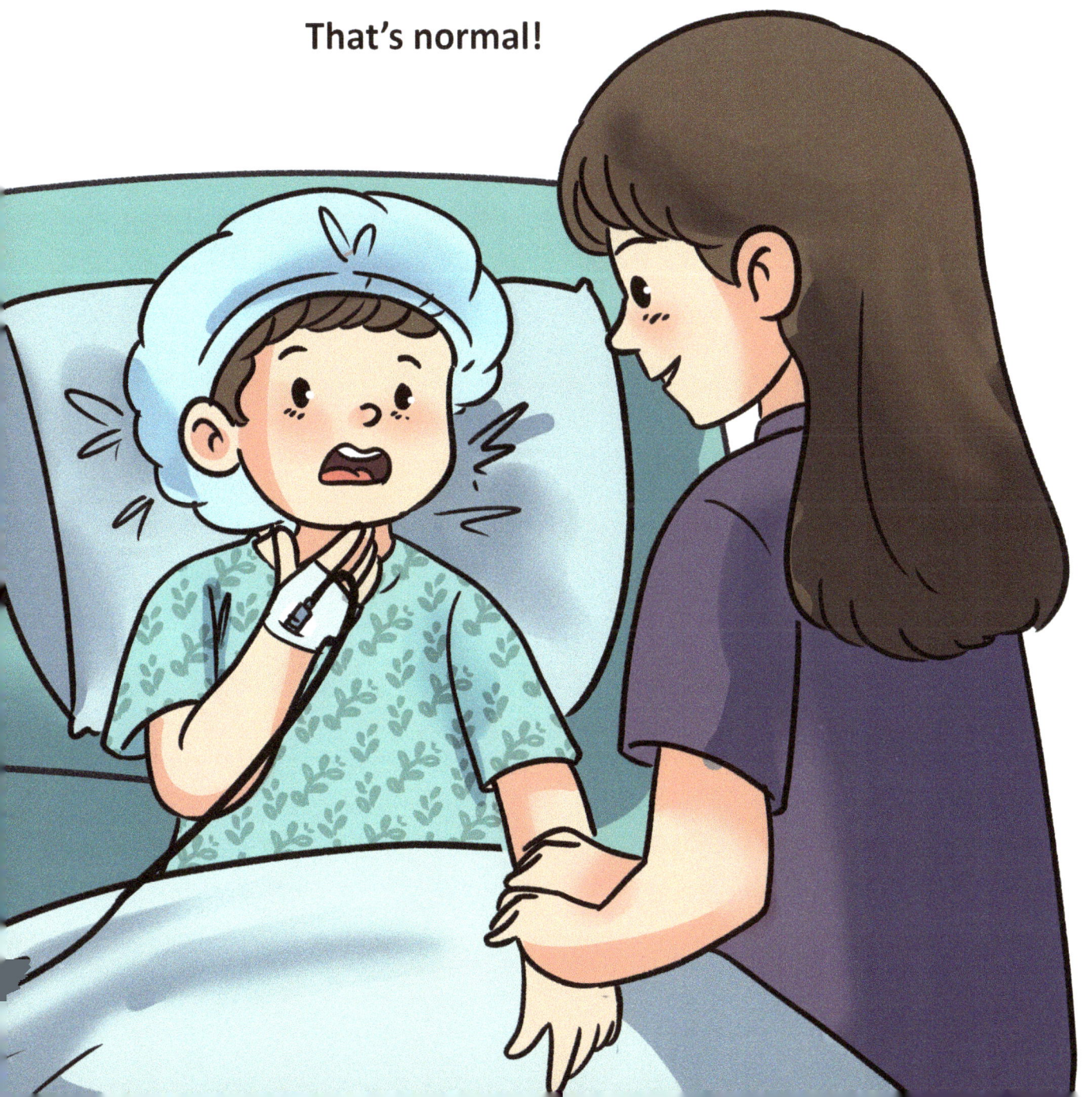

What helps you feel better?
What good ideas do you have?
Place a checkmark (✓) next to your favorites!

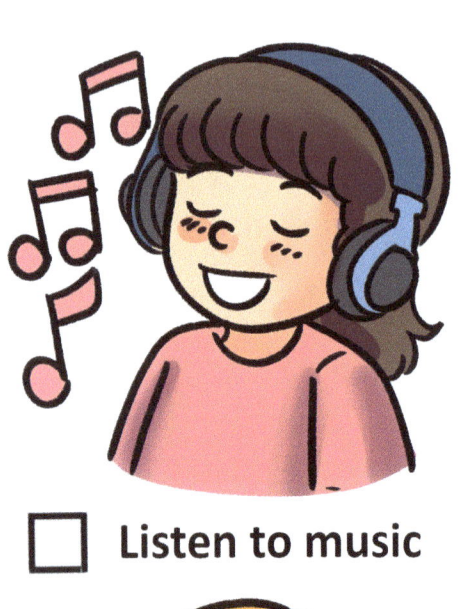

☐ **Listen to music**

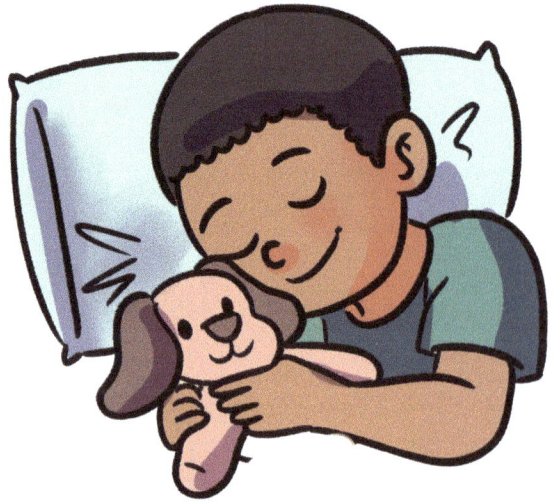

☐ **Rest or take a nap**

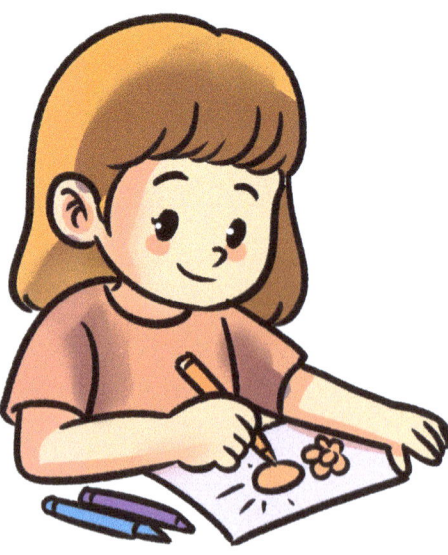

☐ **Color or draw**

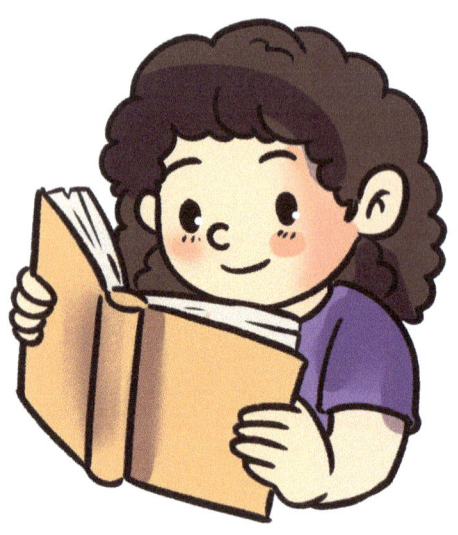

☐ **Read a book**

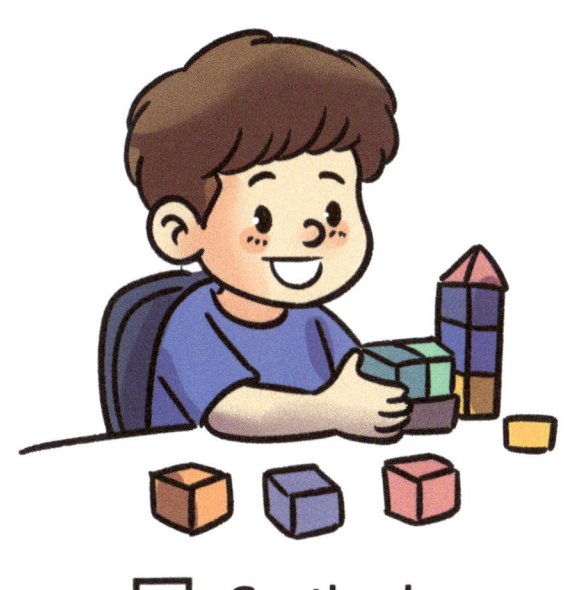
☐ Gentle play

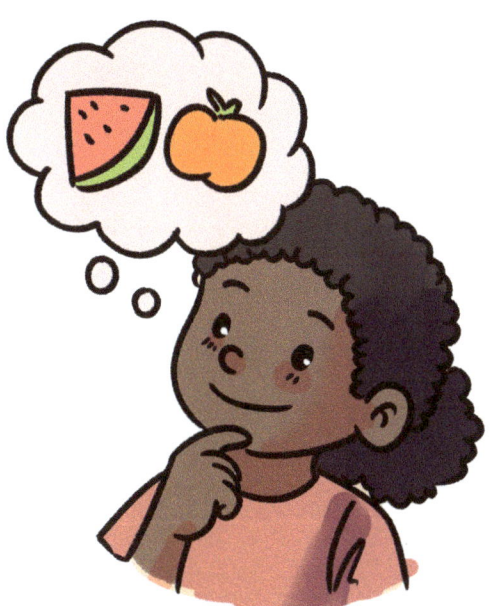
☐ Think about your favorite foods

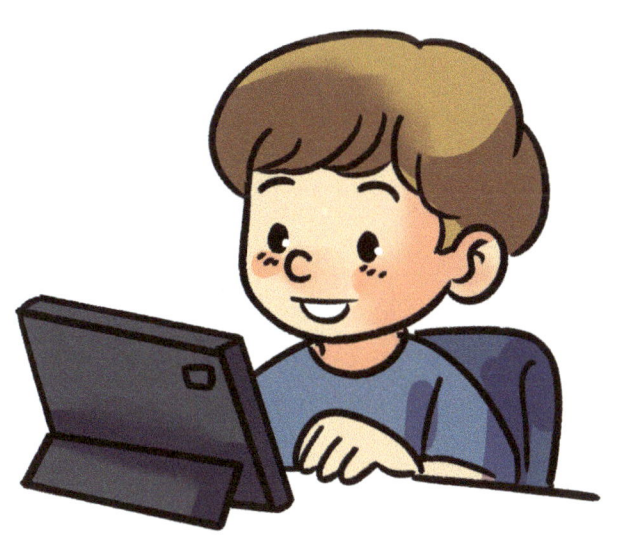
☐ Watch your favorite shows

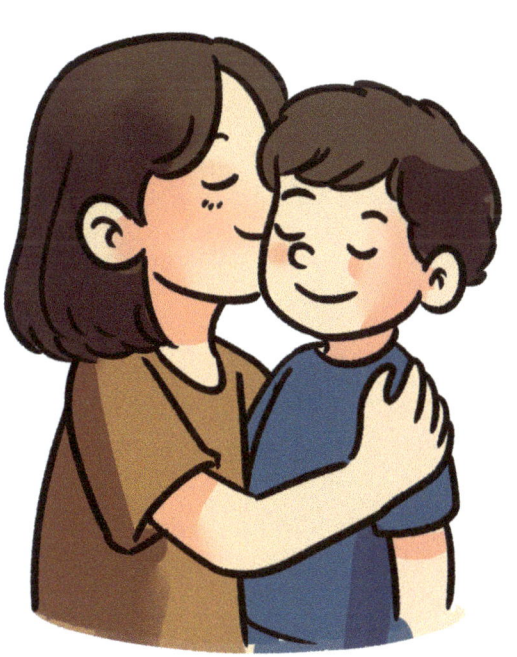
☐ Get a sweet kiss or hug

What will you do after your endoscopy?

A party? A celebration?

What's your favorite way to celebrate?

Draw or write your party plan below.

Speedy recovery!

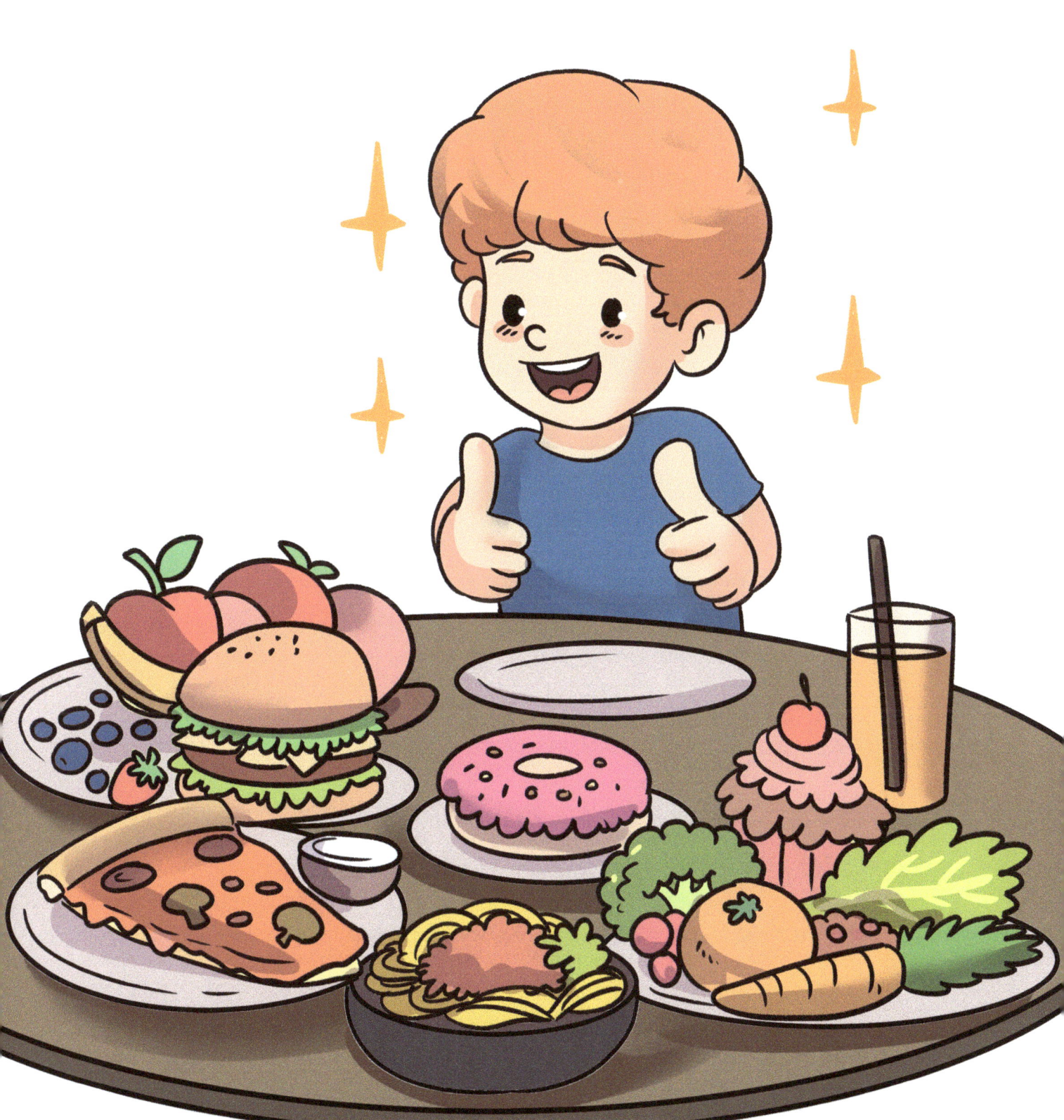

Notes for Parent/Guardian

• In young children, placement of the intravenous (IV) catheter is often done after your child is asleep in the procedure room.

• After the procedure, it is common for children to feel confused, disoriented, or irritable as the anesthesia wears off. Some children may cry, sob, kick, scream, or thrash around. This reaction is normal and usually improves within about one hour.

• Post-procedure instructions and restrictions:
Your child's doctor should give you specific instructions about what your child can and cannot do during the recovery period, how long any activity restrictions should last, and whether follow-up appointments are needed. You should also be told what symptoms to watch for and when to bring your child back to the hospital in case of an emergency. If this information is not discussed, please remind the care team and be sure to receive these instructions before leaving the hospital.

Disclaimer

Please note that the illustrations in this book are not drawn to scale.

This book is written for informational and educational purposes only and is not intended to replace medical advice, diagnosis, or treatment.

Please consult your child's doctor if your child needs medical attention and to confirm that the information in this book applies to your child's specific medical condition and needs. Every child's experience is different, and what your child experiences may not be exactly the same as what is described in this book.

The author and publisher are not responsible, either directly or indirectly, for any damages, monetary losses, or other consequences resulting from the use of information in this book. By reading this book, the reader agrees not to hold the author or publisher responsible for any losses resulting from errors, inaccuracies, or omissions.

Please keep in mind that your child's experience may vary depending on the location, medical facility, healthcare team, and individual medical needs. This book should be used as a supportive resource alongside guidance from your child's doctor.

Thank you.

Did this picture book help your child in some way?
If so, I would love to hear about it!

www.amazon.com/gp/product-review/B0GK6GJJ18

For other book titles, please visit:

www.fzwbooks.com

Connect with the author

email: books@fzwbooks.com
facebook/instagram: @FZWbooks

Books by the author

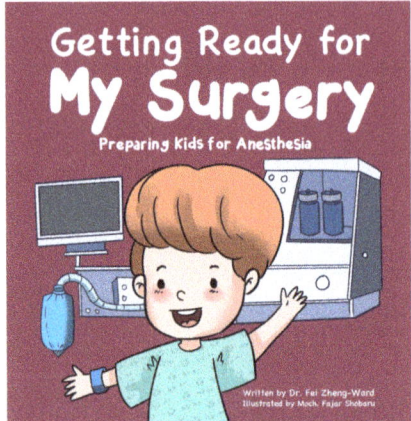
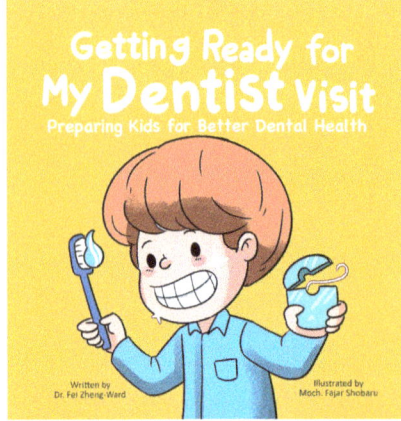
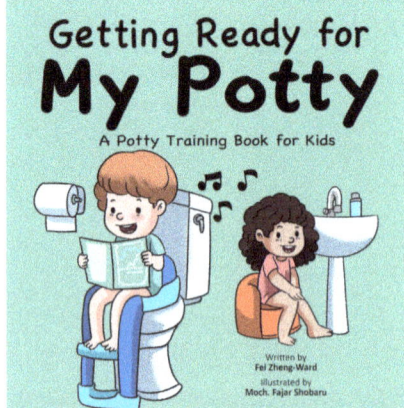
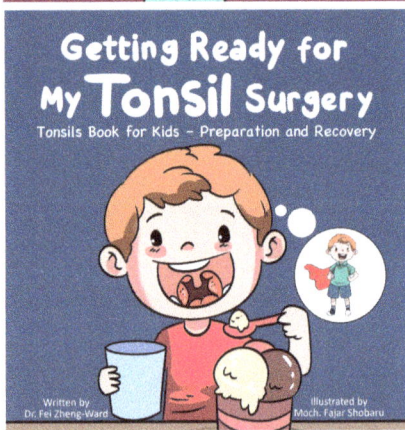
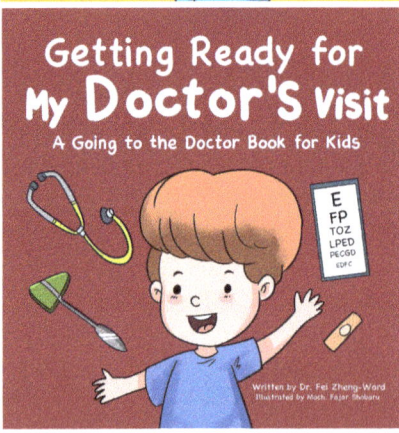
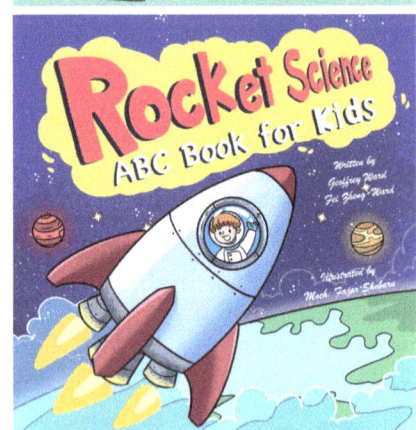
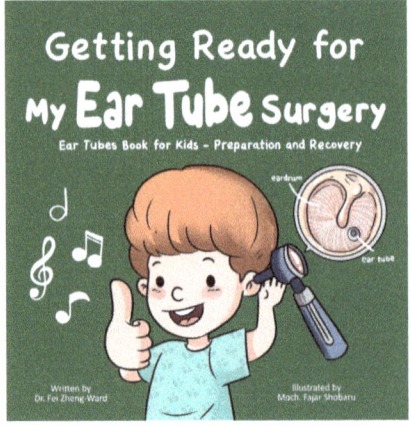
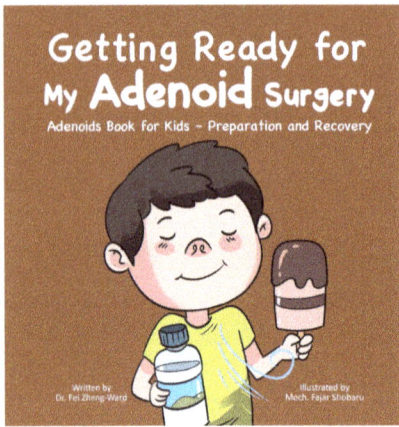
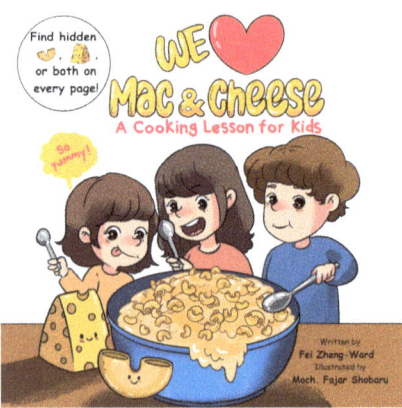

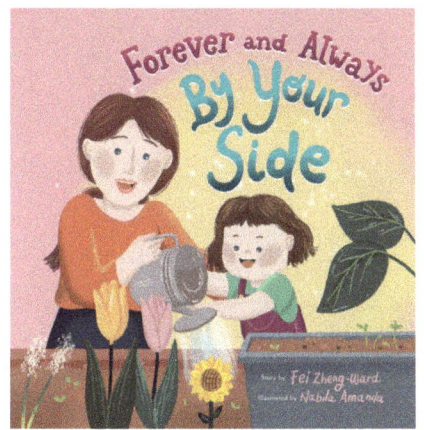
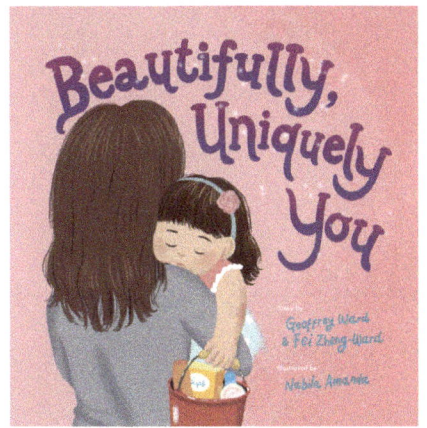
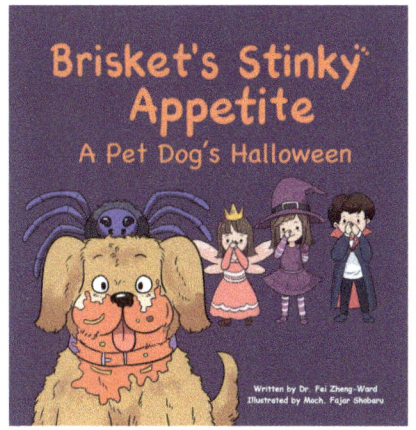
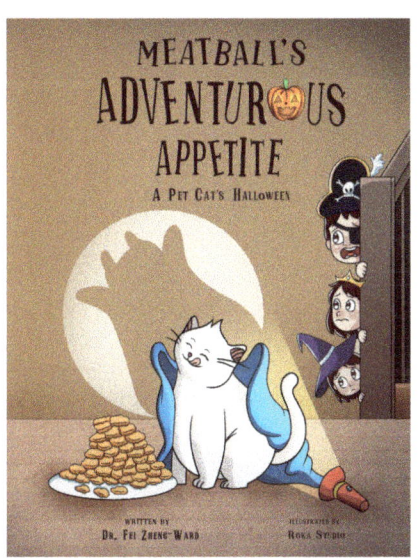
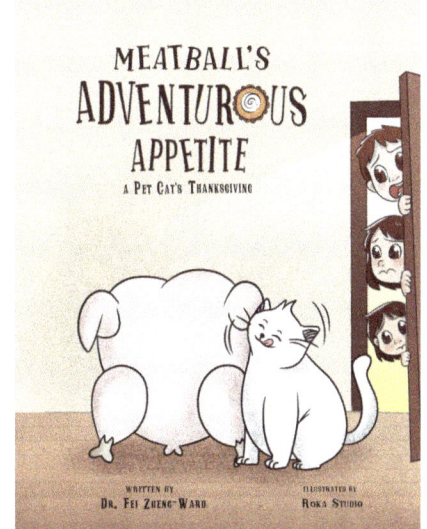
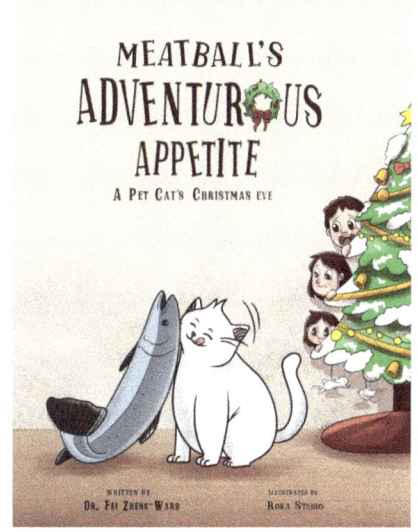
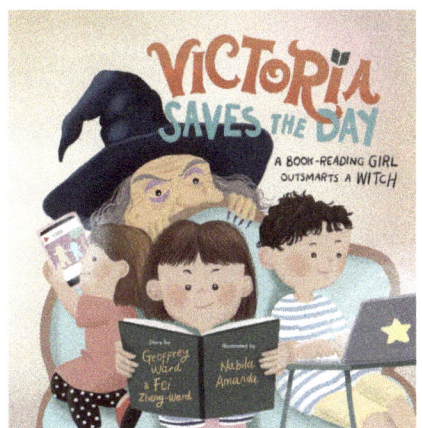
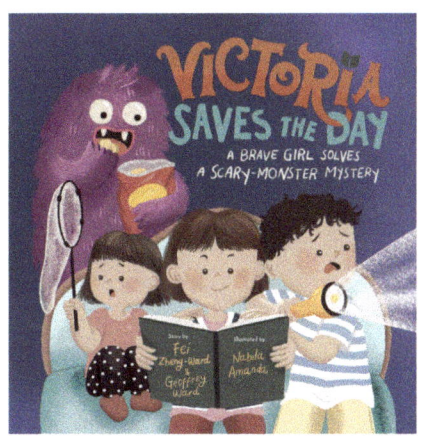
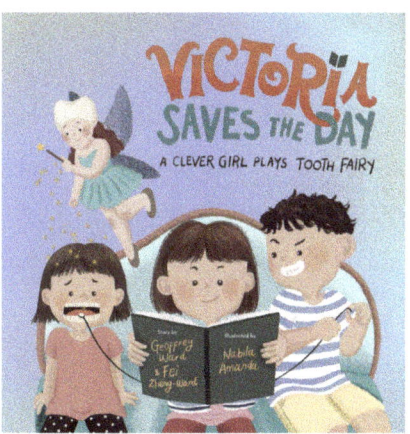

www.ingramcontent.com/pod-product-compliance
Lightning Source LLC
Chambersburg PA
CBHW040002040426
42337CB00032B/5191